HUMAN BODY
Preschool Activity Book

 HANDS-ON LEARNING FOR AGES 3 TO 5

Mazes, Coloring, Connect the Dots, and More!

Kristie Wagner

ROCKRIDGE
PRESS

For my sons— always explore!

NOTE TO CAREGIVERS

Welcome to the *Human Body Preschool Activity Book!*

My name is Kristie Wagner and I've been teaching science in grades 6 through 12 since 2014, but I've noticed that an interest in science starts long before kids get to middle school. Teaching science to young children is important. It helps shape how they approach science later in school and life, but it can be boring if not done correctly. When you introduce science to a child in a fun, interactive way that is developmentally appropriate, you will keep that child interested and wanting to learn more.

In preschool, kids learn to identify colors, shapes, and patterns. They also learn how to follow simple instructions and be creative. This activity book lets kids practice these skills while learning basic facts about human anatomy. Anatomy is great for kids. Most of them are fascinated with the human body—they each have one, after all!

In this book, your preschooler will learn about the brain, nerves, bones, muscles, lungs, heart, digestion, and the immune system. Dozens of fun activities like connect the dots, mazes, color-by-number, and more will engage and entertain while teaching simple concepts about each body system. The activities can be done in order, or your child can jump around as they please, to make learning fun. When they choose an activity, first read the information at the top of the page out loud. It is my hope that their excitement with the topic will stay with them long after they finish this book and that they will, in turn, be curious about other types of science.

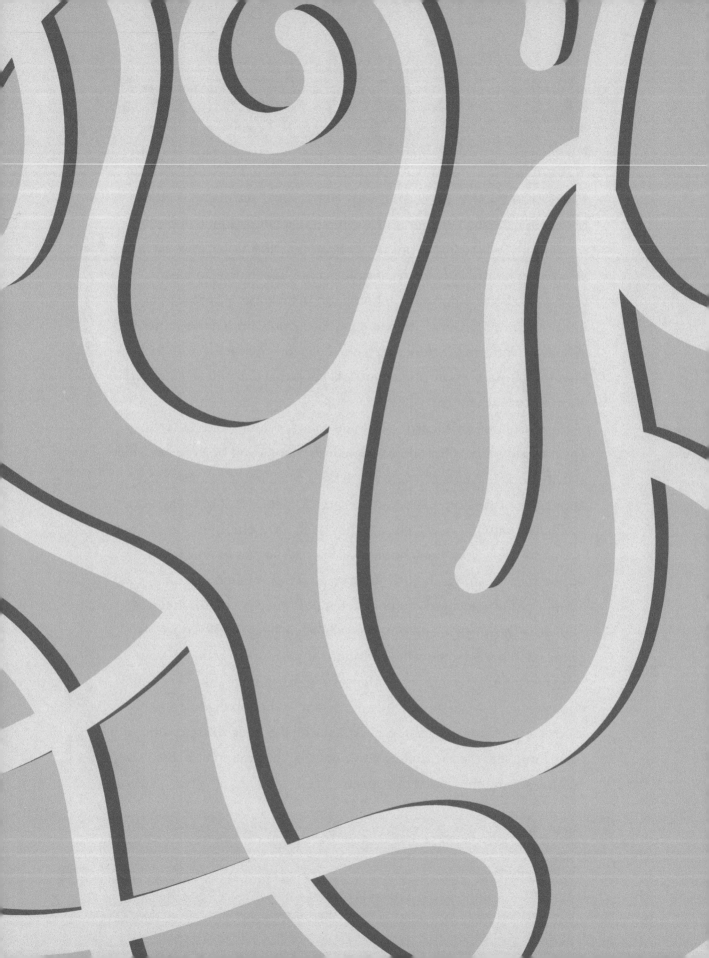

Your Amazing Body

Your body is like a machine with many different parts. Bones, muscles, your heart, and your brain help you move and play every single day! *Follow the key to color in the picture.*

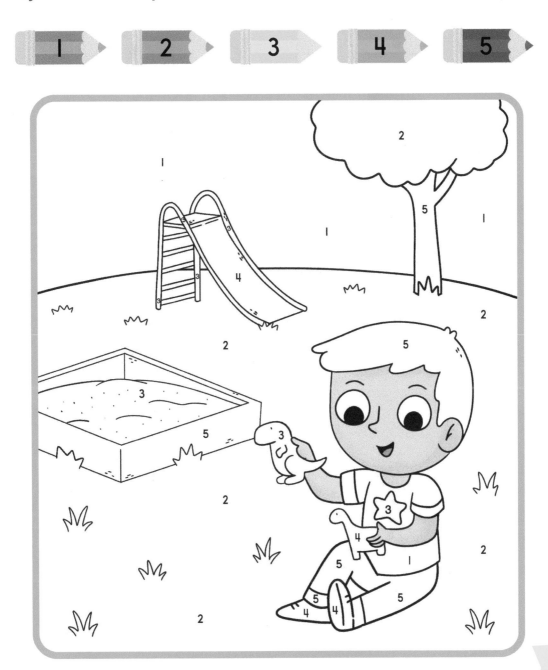

Your Outsides

Your body's inside and outside look very different. Some things you can see on the outside are your eyes, mouth, and ears. *Circle the body parts that you can see when you look in the mirror!*

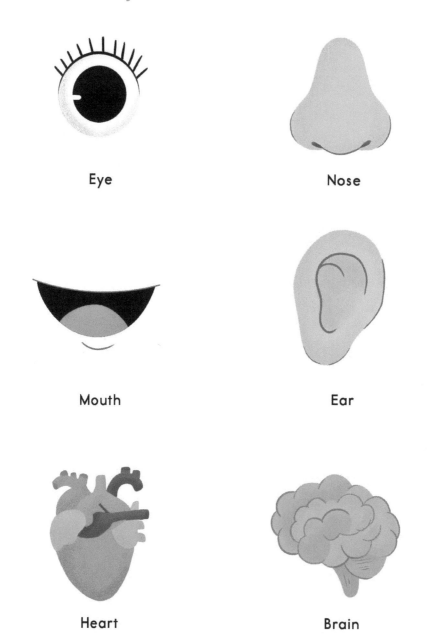

Eye

Nose

Mouth

Ear

Heart

Brain

Your Insides

The inside of your body can only be seen with special machines. That is where your organs and skeleton are. The heart, stomach, and intestines are all organs. *Use your crayons to color this kid's organs.*

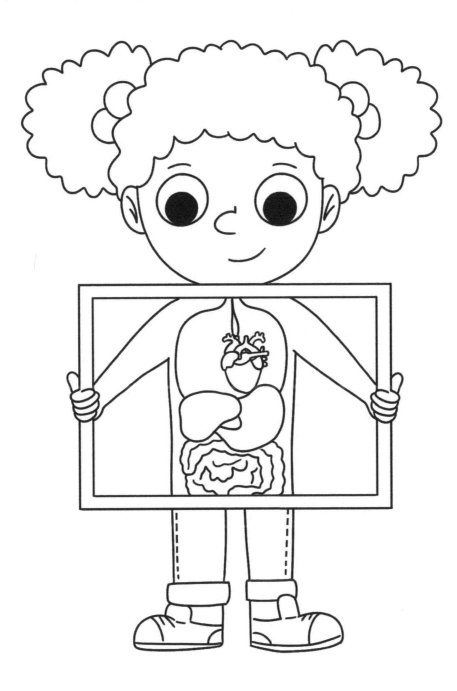

Your Largest Organ

Your largest organ is outside your body. It's your skin! It protects your body from things that do not belong inside it, like germs and dirt. Your skin also makes sure your body is not too cold or too hot. *Connect the dots to see where your skin is the thickest!*

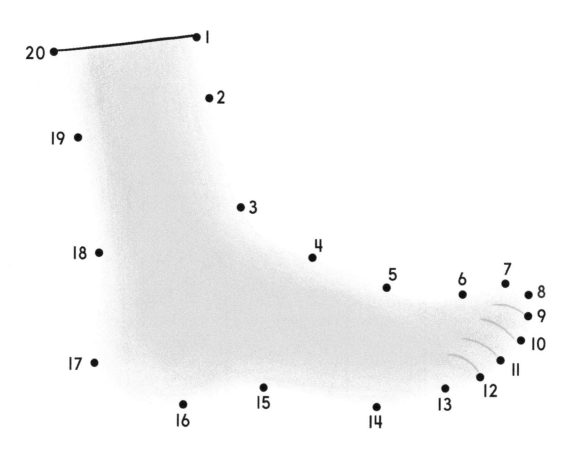

Fascinating Fingerprints!

Fingerprints are tiny grooves in the skin of your fingertips. They help you pick up and hold objects. No two people have the same fingerprints. *Find your way through this fingerprint maze!*

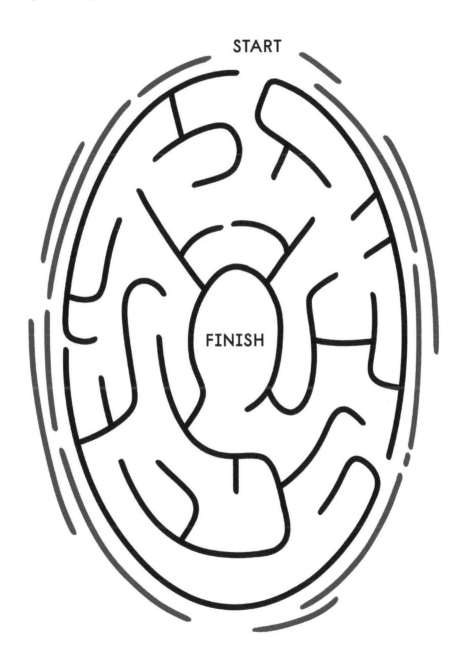

START

FINISH

Super Cells!

The tiniest parts of your body are cells. Different cells make up different body parts. There are bone cells, muscle cells, brain cells, blood cells, and many more. *Circle the cell that comes next in each pattern.*

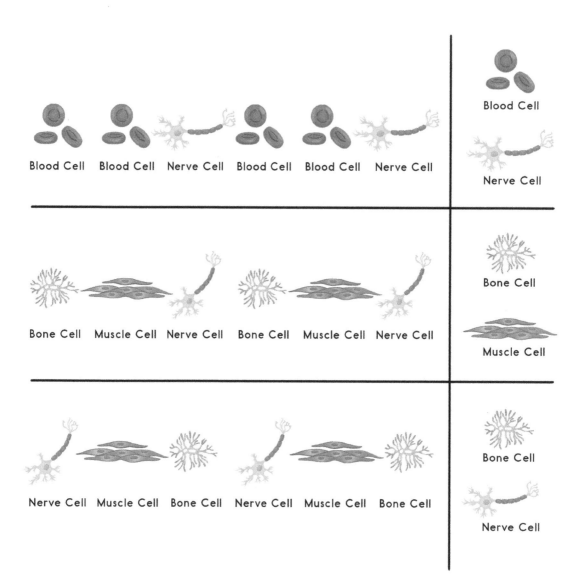

What's That Smell?

Sniff, sniff! When you smell something with your nose, tiny scent particles are sucked inside. Your brain figures out what those particles are and tells you what you smelled! *Circle the things that smell good to you.*

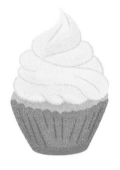

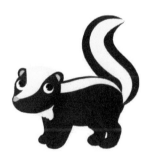

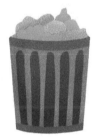

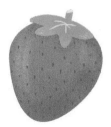

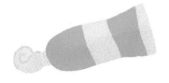

Water Body

Your body may feel solid, but it is about 60 percent water. That is more than half! Your lungs are made of the most water and your bones are made of the least. A jellyfish is almost all water! *Follow the key to color this watery scene.*

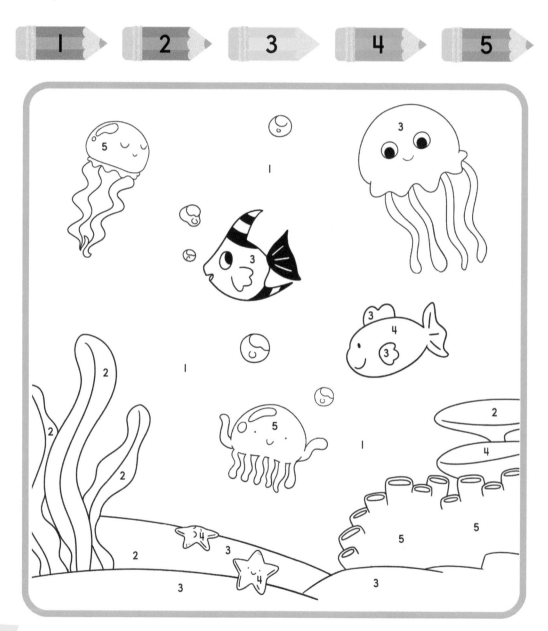

Tasty Snacks

Your tongue is covered with tiny bumps called taste buds. They send messages to your brain when you eat something. Then your brain figures out if what you ate tasted salty, sweet, sour, or bitter. *Circle the snack that is different.*

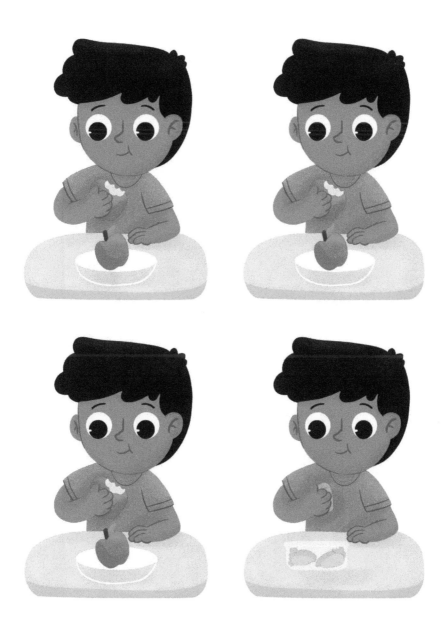

Eye See

When you look at something, your eyes actually view it upside down. Your brain gets the picture from your eyes, and it turns the scene right-side up! *Complete each pattern by picking the next eye.*

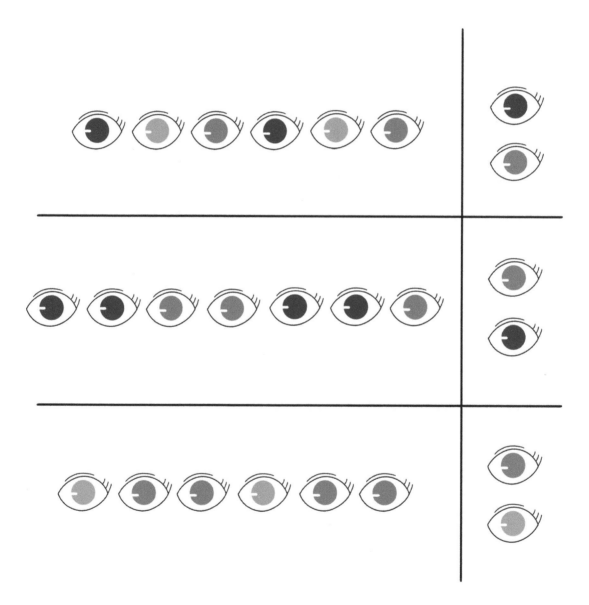

Something Soft

- - - - - - - - - - - - - - -

Your skin is able to feel if something is sharp, rough, sticky, or soft. It can also tell if something is wet, dry, hot, or cold. *Connect the dots to see something that feels soft!*

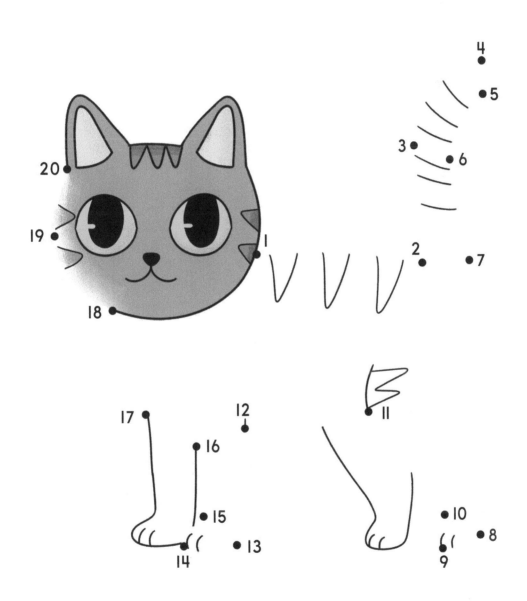

How You Hear

When you hear something, the sound goes in your ear. The sound makes parts inside your ear move. Your brain reads these movements and figures out what you heard. *Finish the picture to see an animal with big ears (to hear with!).*

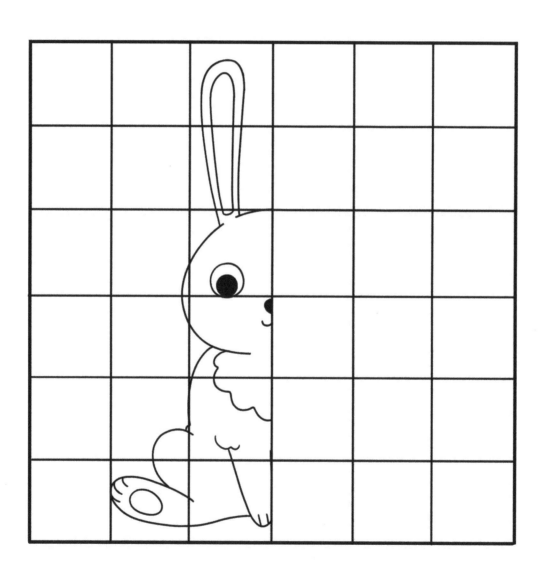

Your Brain and Nerves

Your nervous system is made up of your brain, spinal cord, and nerves. Your nerves take messages from your body to the spinal cord. The messages travel up the spinal cord to the brain. *Color this picture of the nervous system. Use a different color for the brain.*

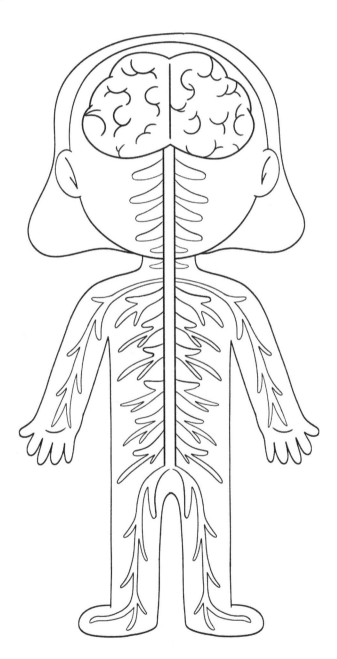

Think about It!

Your brain is in charge of your entire body. You need to tell your brain to make some things happen, like talking. Your brain controls other things, like breathing, without you needing to think about them! *You will need to use your brain to finish this picture!*

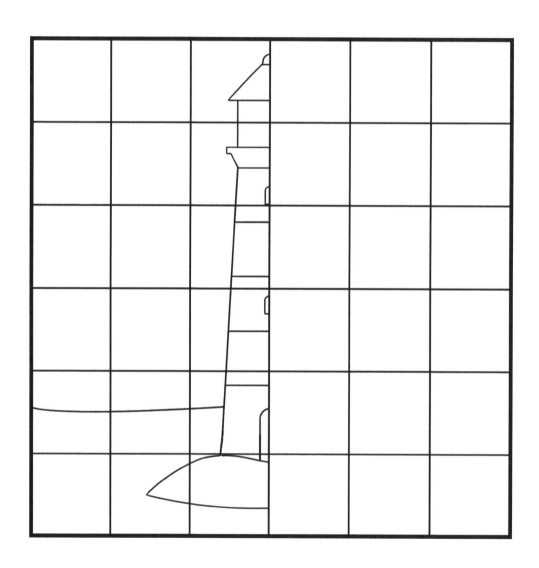

Speedy Delivery!

Your nerves deliver messages from your brain to your other body parts. For example, when you want to walk, nerves deliver directions to the muscles in your legs. These messages travel faster than a race car! *Complete the maze to get the race car to the finish line.*

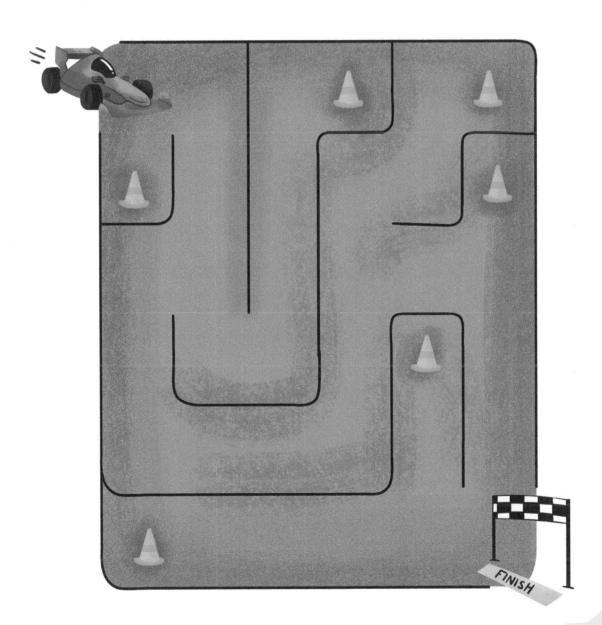

15

Command Central

When you touch, smell, hear, or see, different nerves send messages to your brain. Then your brain tells your body what to do in return. When you feel something cold, your brain can tell you to shiver to warm up. *Circle the picture of fun in the cold that is different from the others!*

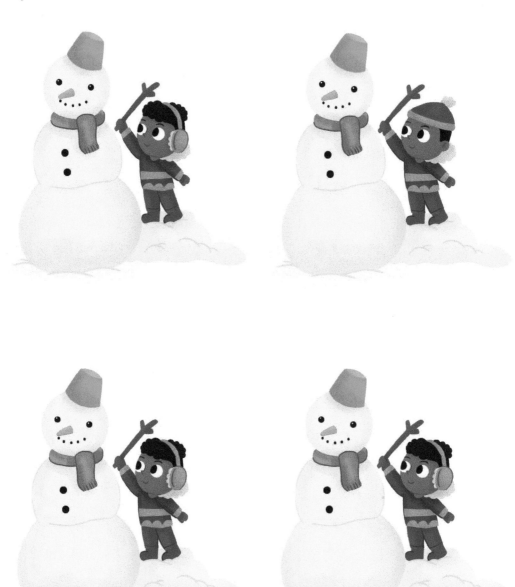

Memory Keeper

The different sections of your brain, called lobes, are in charge of different things. Learning and memory are the temporal lobe's job. **Complete the patterns by circling what comes next.**

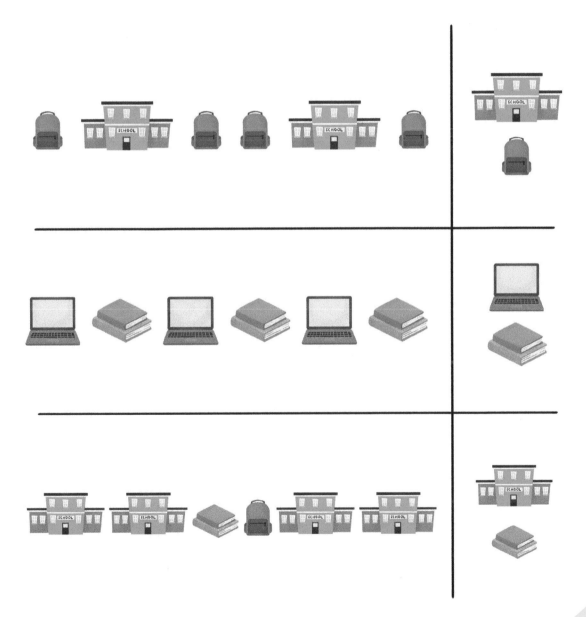

Make a Face

Your brain controls your feelings. It tells you when to feel happy, sad, angry, or scared. Something called the limbic system in your brain controls them. *Circle all the things that make you feel happy!*

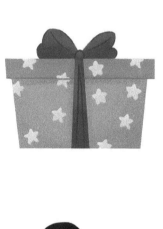

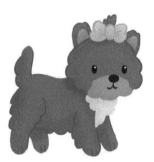

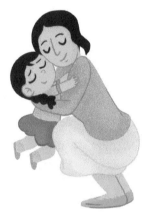

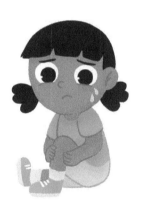

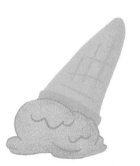

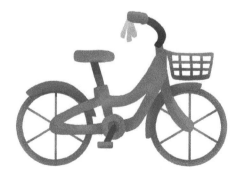

Your Bones

Your bones come in all shapes and sizes. All your bones together form your skeleton. Your skeleton gives your body its shape, protects your organs, and lets you move. *Connect the dots to finish the skeleton!*

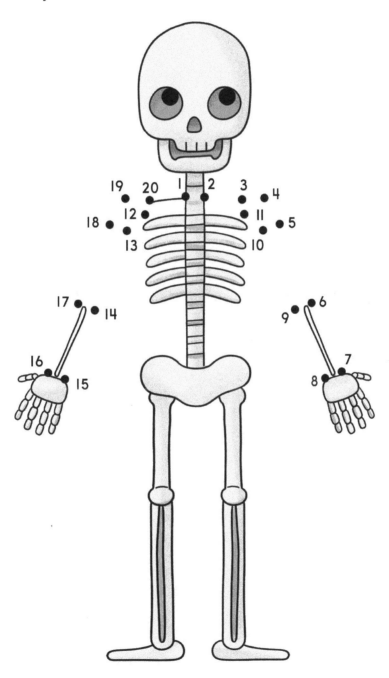

What's In Your Head?

Your skull protects one of your most important organs—your brain. The skull is not one bone. It is made of 22 bones. *Finish the picture of the skull.*

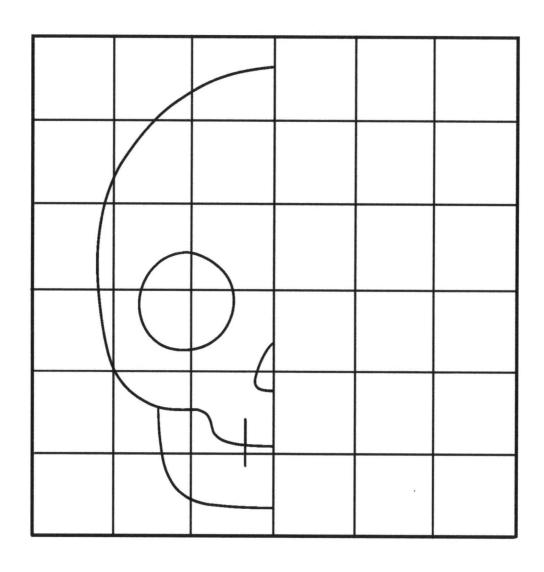

Long Leg Bones

Leg bones are big and strong. They have to be since your whole body sits on top of them! Your upper leg bone is called a femur. It the longest bone in your body! *Circle all the animals with legs.*

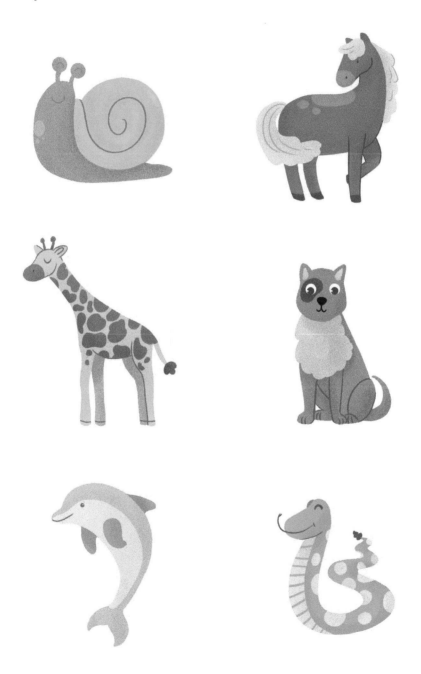

There's a What In My Ear?

The smallest bones in your body are inside your ears. They vibrate, or move, when sound enters your ears. The brain uses those vibrations to figure out what you are hearing. The outside of your ear is made of cartilage—a rubbery, bendy tissue. *Connect the dots to give this elephant its ears!*

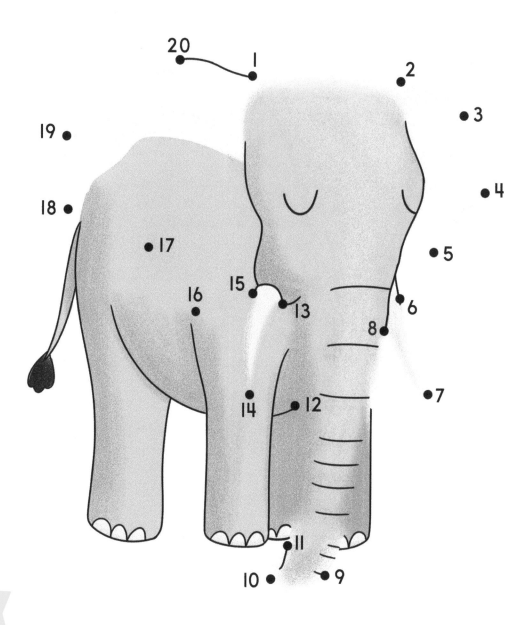

Being Bendy

Your joints are the places where two bones meet. Without them, you could not bend or move. Joints let you walk, throw a ball, talk, and even dance.

Circle the dancing ballerina who is different from the rest.

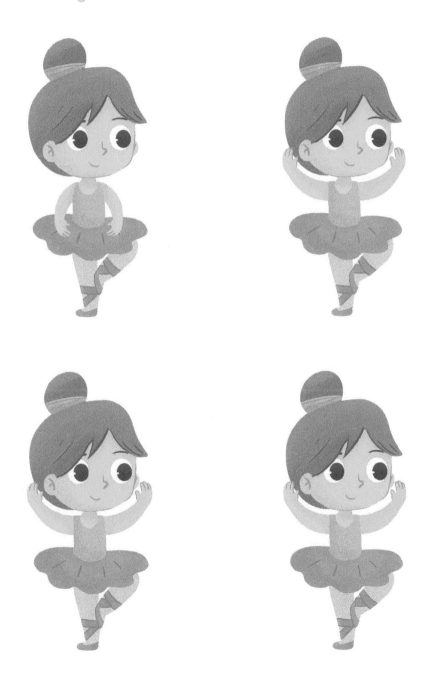

Helping You Heal

Sometimes a bone breaks. When this happens, your body makes new bone cells to repair the break. A doctor puts a cast on it to protect the bone while it heals. *Help this child get to the doctor to take their cast off!*

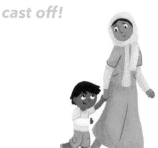

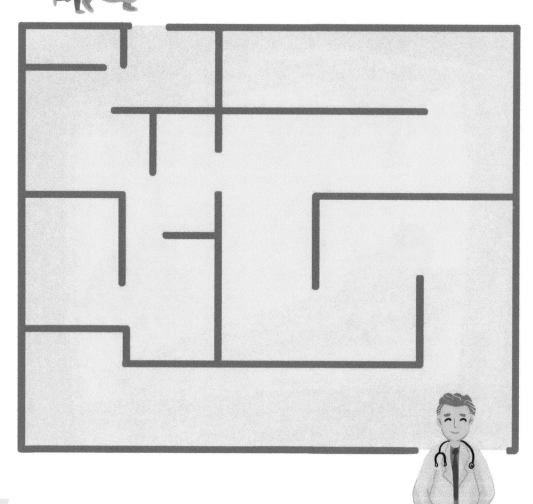

Your Muscles

Your skeleton can't move on its own. It needs muscles to do that! Many different muscles are attached to your bones. *Color this picture of a kid showing you their muscles!*

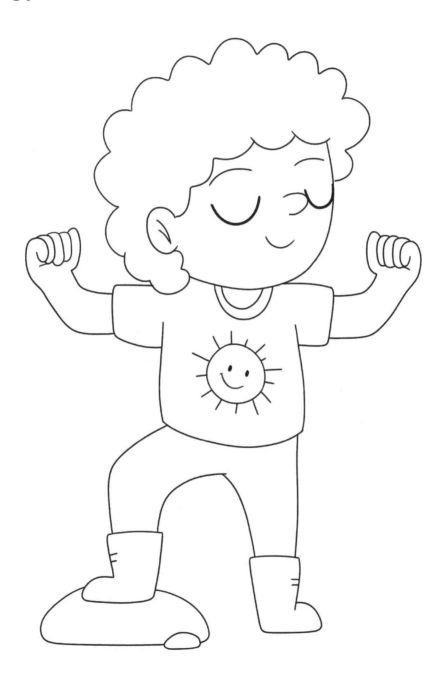

Move It!

Different types of muscles do different things. Muscles help digest your food, pump your heart, make you breathe, and move your body. *Circle the kids who are exercising their leg muscles.*

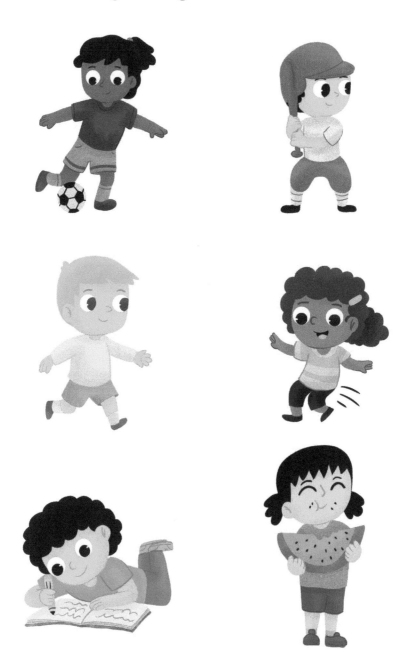

Special Muscles

Your heart is one strong muscle. Every time it beats, the heart muscle squeezes and pushes blood around your body. Your heart is about the size of your fist. *Connect the dots to see the animal with the biggest heart!*

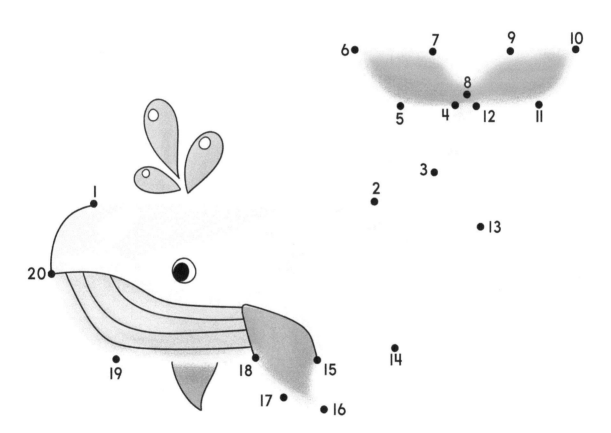

Muscle Teams

Some muscles work together to help you move. In your arms, biceps muscles bend your elbow. Triceps muscles pull your arm straight. *Circle the baseball player who is different from the others.*

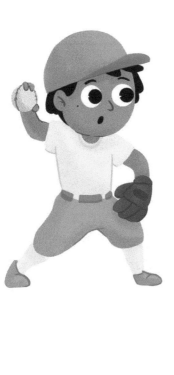 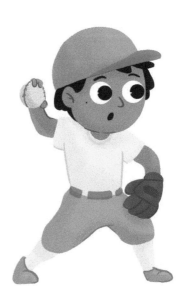

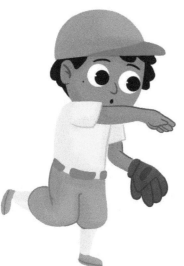 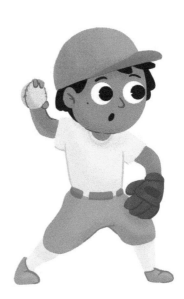

Always Moving

Your heart, diaphragm (your breathing muscle), and the muscles in your stomach and intestines work on their own without you thinking about them. Put your hand on your chest to feel your heart beating now. *Then complete the patterns by circling the next heart!*

Your Beautiful Smile

Did you know your face has 42 muscles? Those muscles help you smile, frown, or make a funny face when you smell something icky! Finish the picture. *Then make it a self-portrait by adding your own hairstyle!*

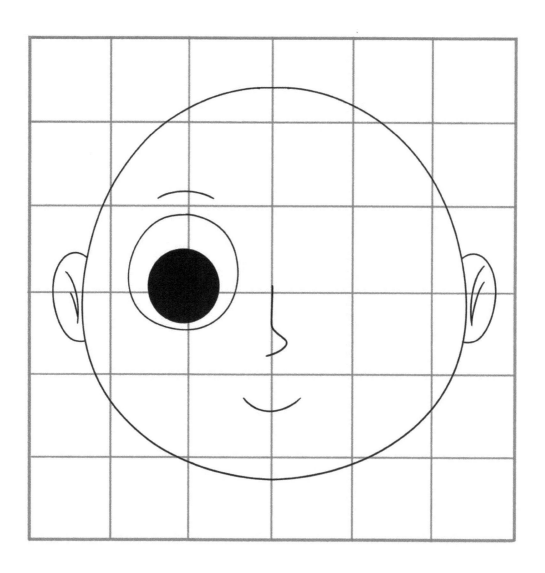

Your Lungs

Your lungs have one of your body's most important jobs—breathing. When you exercise, your breathing speeds up. When you relax, your breathing slows down. *Color this picture of a child doing a breathing exercise.*

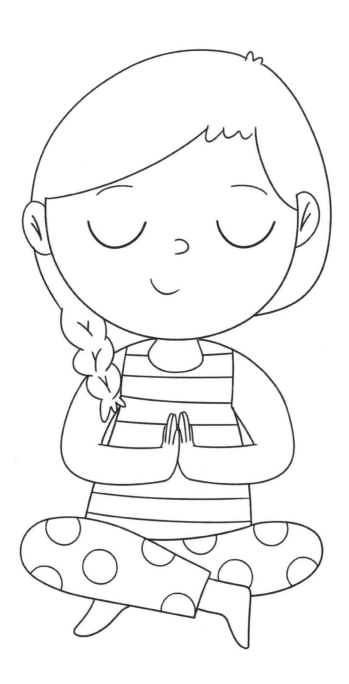

Breathe In

When you breathe in, or inhale, oxygen goes into your lungs. Blood picks up the oxygen and your heart beats to send it to your entire body. When you inhale, you might also smell something. *Complete the maze to find the sweet-smelling flowers!*

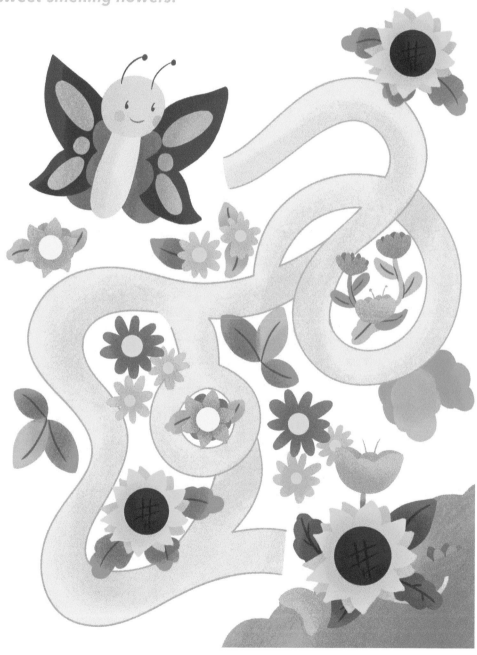

Breathe Out

When you breathe out, or exhale, carbon dioxide leaves your lungs. Carbon dioxide is a gas that doesn't help your body, but it does help trees and other plants. Finish the picture of the tree. *Add as many apples as you'd like!*

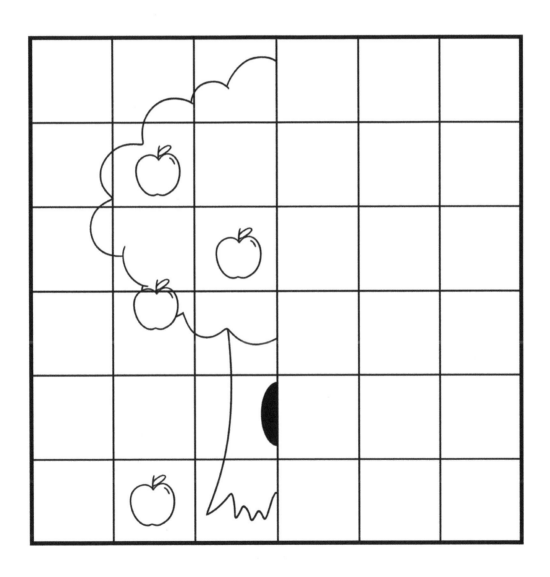

Breathing Buddy

Breathing can be hard work! A muscle, called the diaphragm, makes your lungs fill with air when you breathe in and pushes the air back out when you breathe out. *Connect the dots to see what the diaphragm can do.*

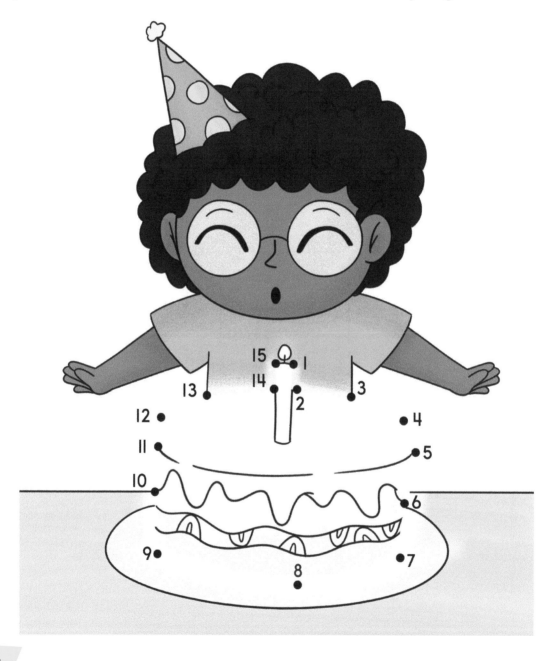

Made You Yawn!

When you are tired, sometimes your body makes you yawn. When you yawn, you take a biiiig long breath of lots of air. *Circle the bedtime scene that's different from the others. Did you yawn?*

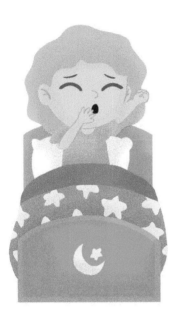 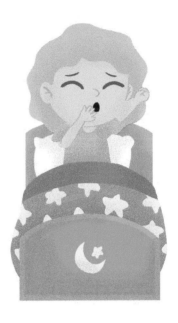

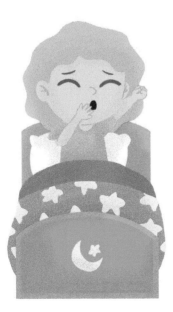 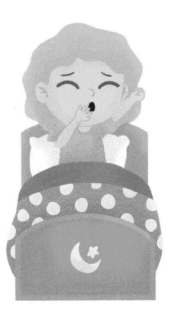

Laughing Lungs

Without your lungs, you wouldn't be able to live. You also wouldn't be able to talk, sing, hiccup, or laugh. *Connect the dots to find a silly picture to make you giggle!*

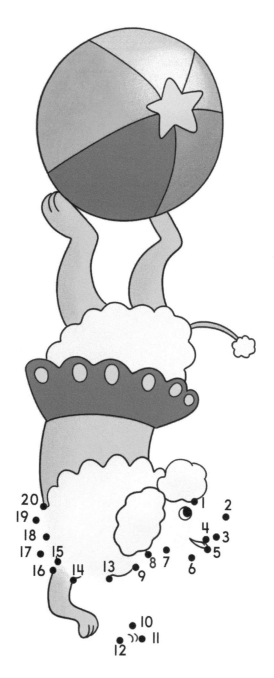

Your Heart

Your heart pumps blood through your entire body. That blood brings oxygen, vitamins, and minerals to every cell. The heart has four sections called chambers. *Use the key to color in the heart's chambers, then use any color for the rest of the heart.*

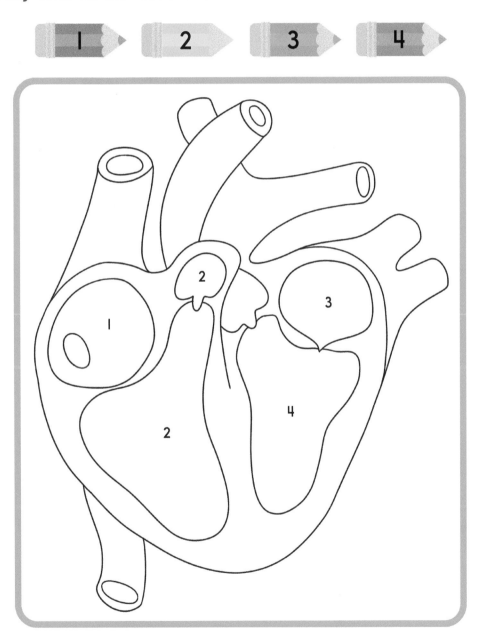

Heart Healthy Choices

Since your heart is a muscle, it needs to stay strong, and you can help it by staying active and eating healthy foods like fruits and vegetables. *Circle the foods that help keep your heart healthy!*

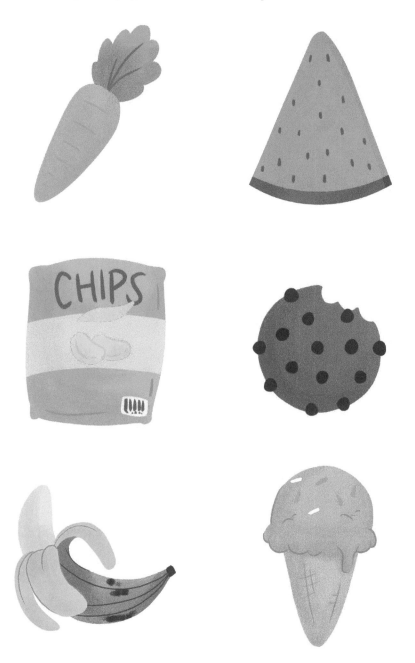

Your Beautiful Blood

Blood is made of plasma (the liquid part), red blood cells, white blood cells, and platelets. Your body is about half water. Most of your blood is made inside your bones. **Complete these patterns by circling the next blood cell.**

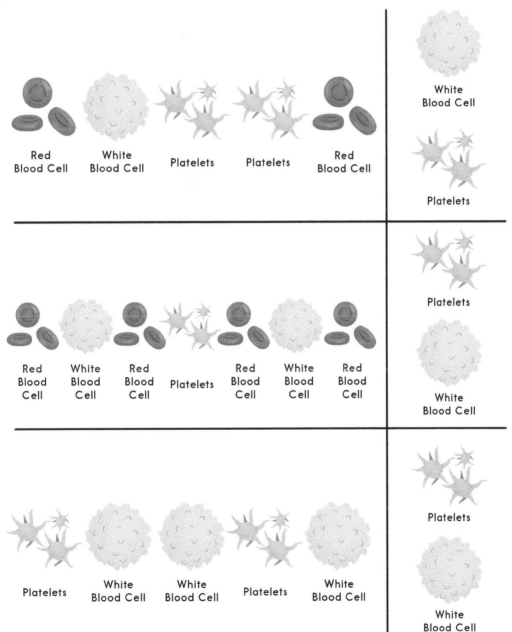

Stop the Bleeding

If you cut yourself, platelets in your blood come to the rescue. They are sticky little cells that clump together to stop the bleeding and help make a scab. Bandages help, too! *Circle the picture that is different.*

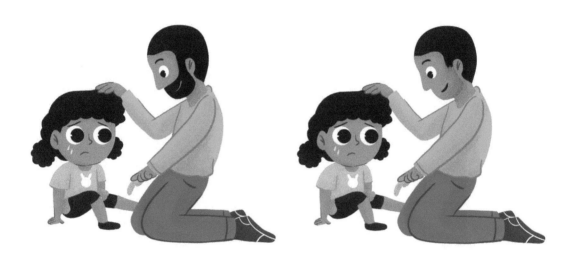

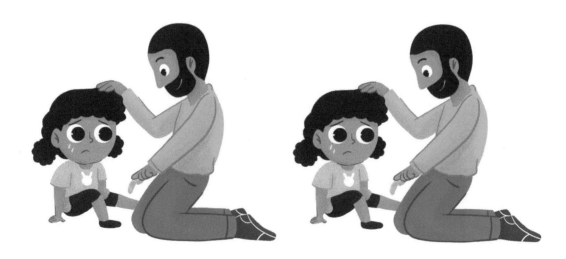

Blood Highways

Blood travels through three different vessels, or tubes, in your body. Blood with oxygen travels in arteries. Blood without oxygen travels in veins. Tiny capillaries connect veins and arteries together. *Finish the maze to help the heart pump blood through the veins to the lungs!*

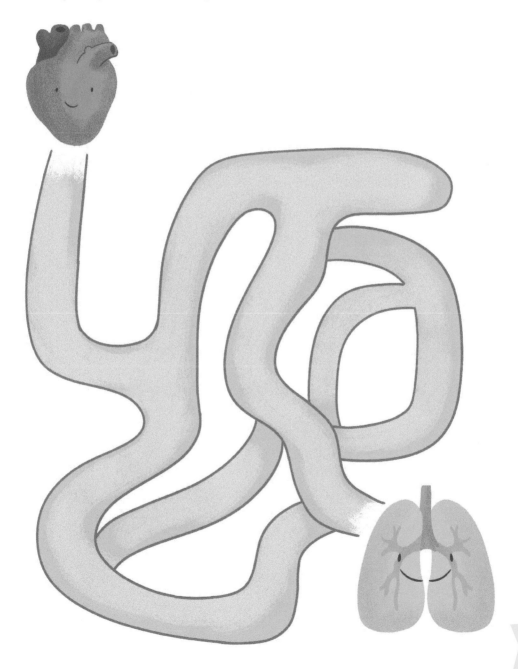

Tiny Carriers

Red blood cells are red. Surprise! Their job is to carry oxygen to all the body's cells and remove carbon dioxide. They are shaped like donuts and make up almost half of your blood! *Circle the objects that are shaped like blood cells—round with empty space inside, like that tasty donut!*

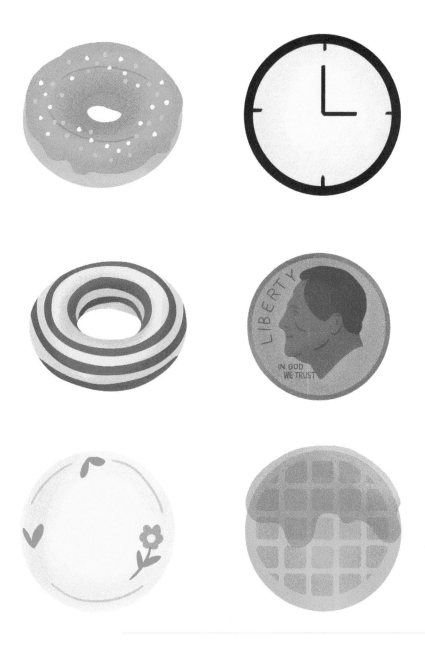

Your Immune System

Your immune system is always on the lookout for germs. When it finds a germ, it sends different kinds of white blood cells to the scene. One type of white blood cell, the macrophage, actually gobbles germs up! *Color the picture to defend the body against germs!*

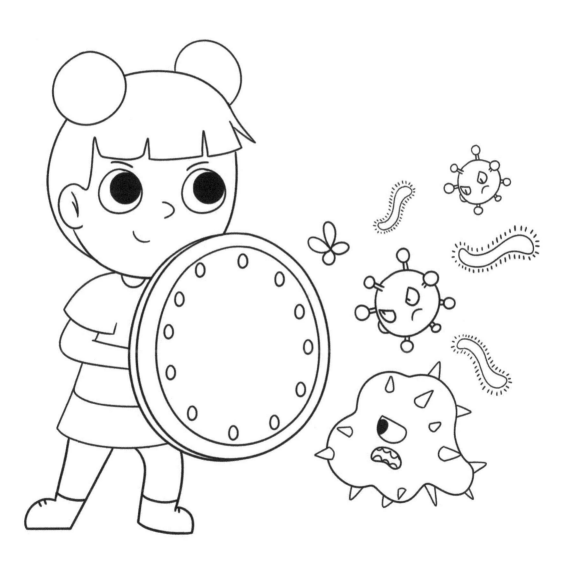

43

Germ Attack

Germs are tiny organisms that can make us sick if they get inside our bodies. Bacteria and viruses are two types of germs. *Complete the germ patterns by circling the next bacteria or virus!*

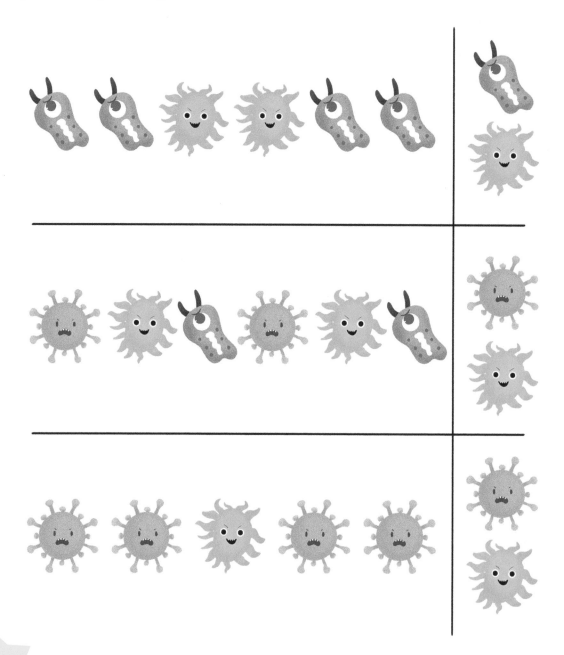

Stop That Germ!

Antibodies help attack the germs that get inside your body so you don't get sick. Doctors use vaccines to help your body make antibodies for germs, like the flu or COVID-19. *Solve the maze to help the vaccine fight the virus.*

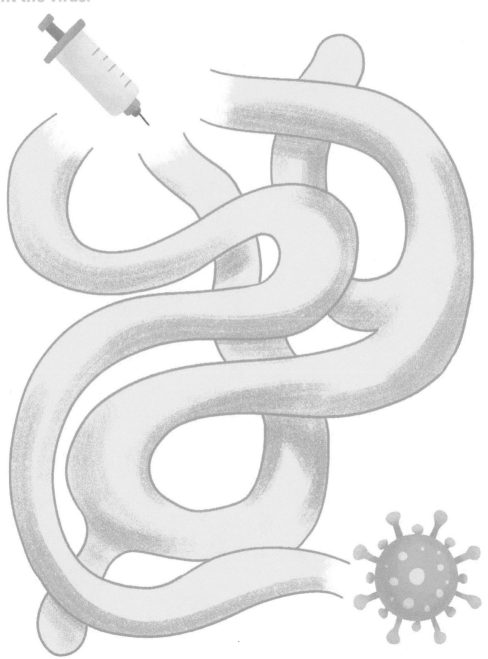

Superhero Snacks

You can eat healthy foods to help your body protect itself against germs. Fruits, vegetables, and almonds help make your immune system strong!

Connect the dots to see a food that can help your immune system.

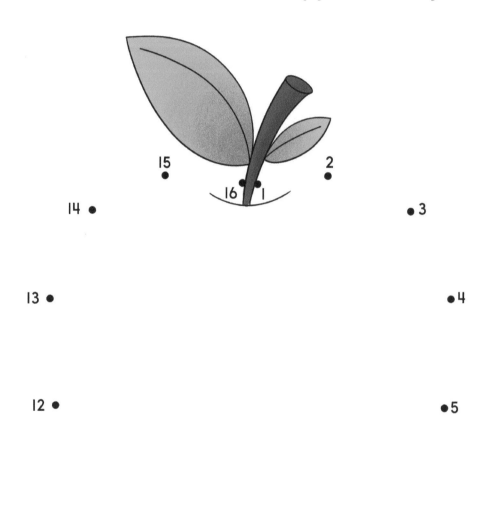

Healthy Habits

You can help your immune system by drinking lots of water, getting enough sleep, and exercising. These are called healthy habits. *Circle all the things that help you have healthy habits.*

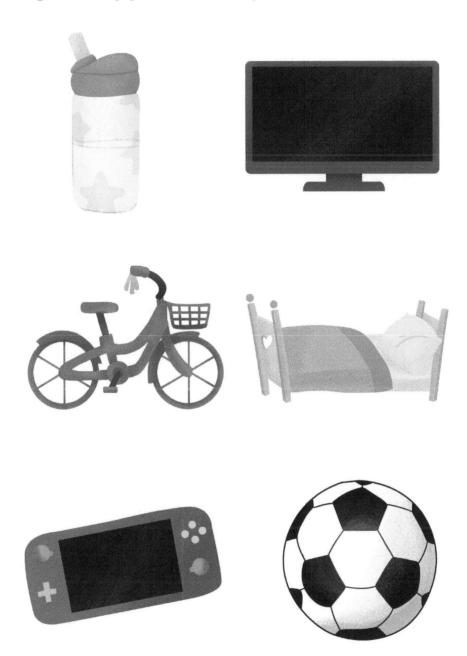

Antibodies in Action

Your tonsils are small organs in the back of your throat. They catch germs and fight them with antibodies. When you get sick, they can swell up and make your throat sore. *Finish the picture to see something that makes you feel better when you have a sore throat.*

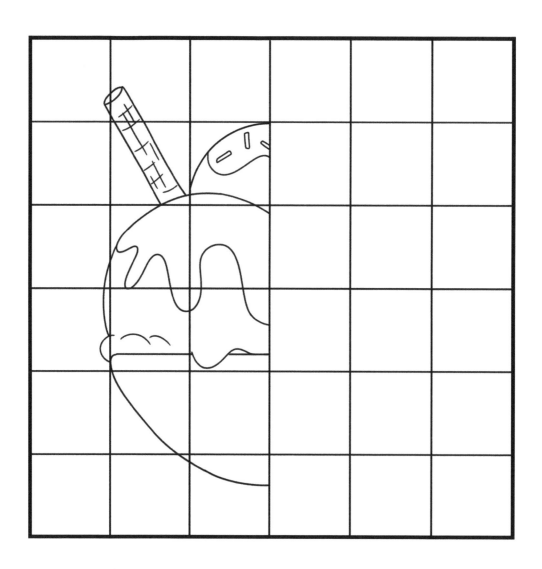

Your Digestive System

Your digestive system helps you get energy from the food that you eat. Digestion starts when you chew your food and ends when you poop.

Color the picture of the kid eating lunch.

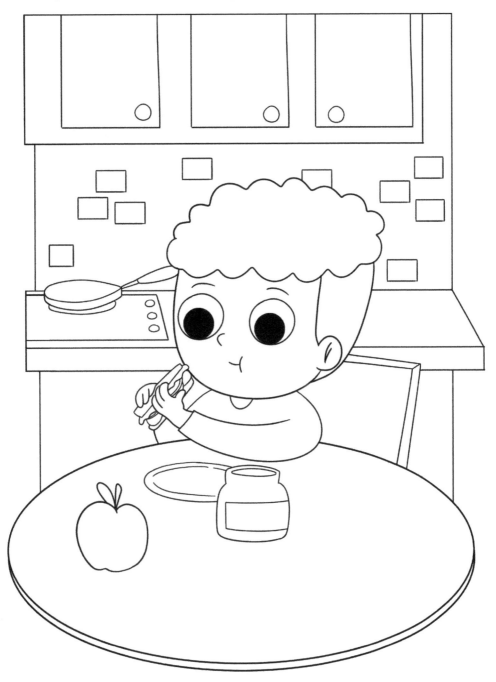

Chew, Chew, Chew!

Make sure you chew your food well! When you chew your food, you start digesting it. Chewing also helps the food move down your esophagus and into your stomach. *Complete the patterns by circling the next food!*

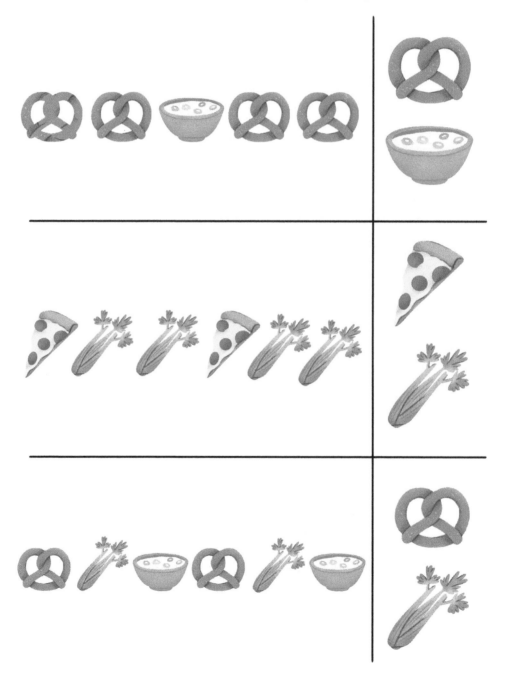

Wash It Down

After you swallow, the food or liquid travels through your esophagus. Your esophagus is a tube made of muscle that squeezes the food down to your stomach. *Circle the picture that is different.*

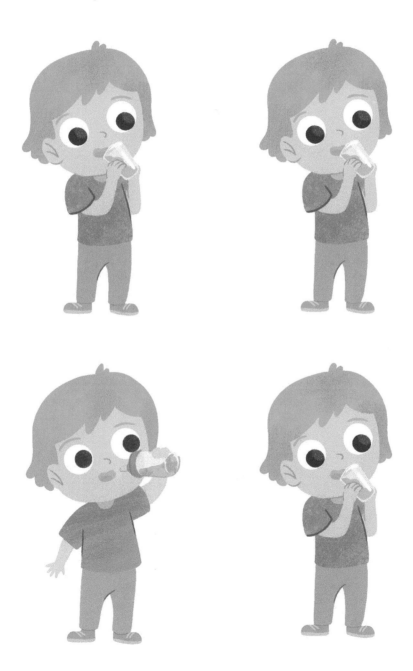

A Full Stomach

Your stomach's job is to make the food you eat into something your body can use. It uses acid and strong muscles to mash and squeeze the food into a soupy mix. *Connect the dots to draw a stomach. Then draw some food inside for it to digest.*

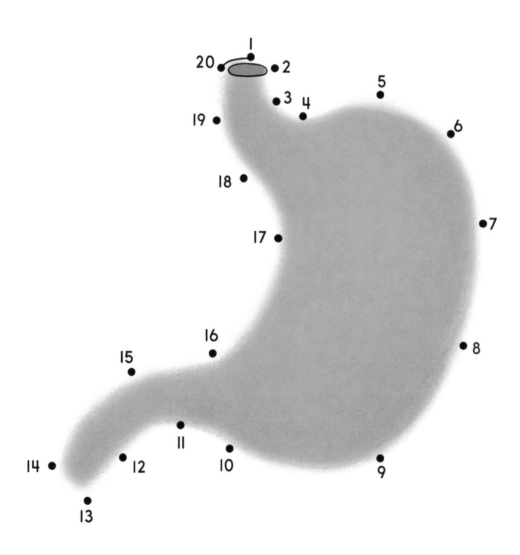

A-maz-ing Intestines!

After your stomach is done with food, the food moves into your intestines. The intestines take out the nutrients—the parts that give you energy—and blood cells pick them up. *Complete the maze to help the tasty treat travel through the intestines.*

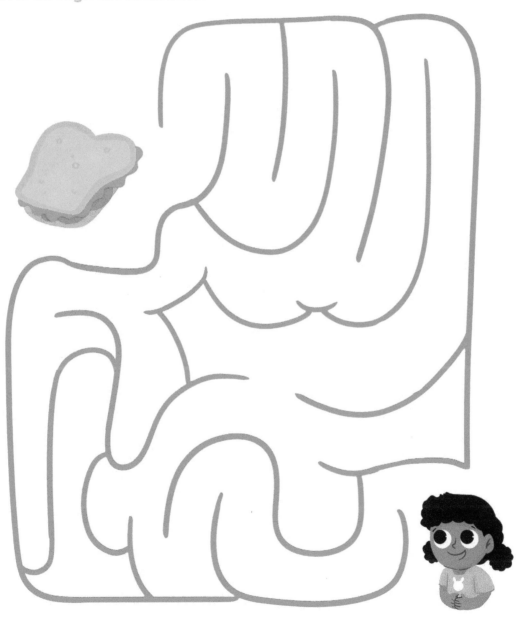

Waste Removal

After your body has taken all the nutrients from the food, it gets rid of the rest as waste—pee or poop. Pee is liquid and leaves through your bladder. Poop is solid and leaves through your anus (your bottom). *Circle the picture that is different.*

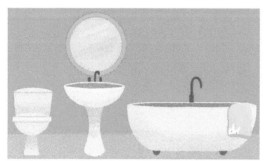

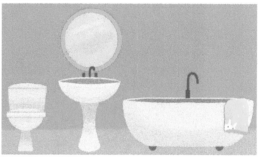

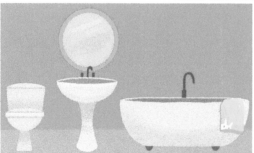

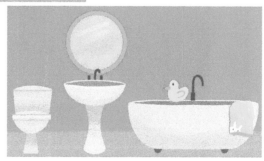

Move It!

Your bones and muscles protect your organs and help you move and grow. Without them, you would have no shape and could not run or play! *Color the picture of kids having fun.*

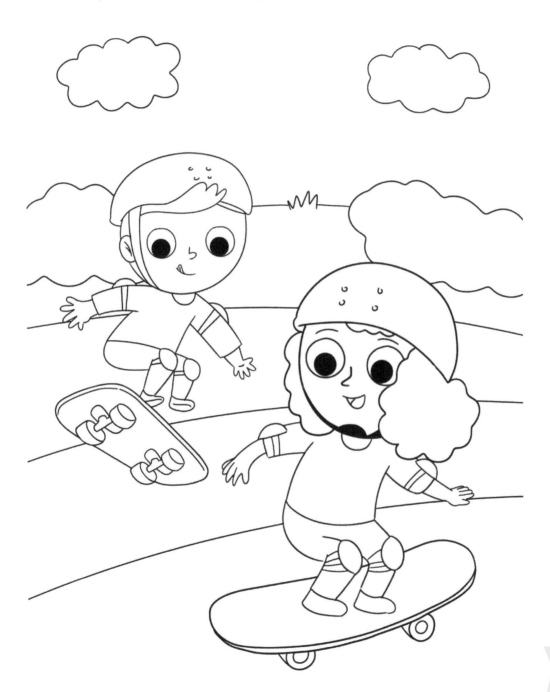

Fuel Up!

Your digestive system helps you get energy and nutrients from the food you eat. Food also helps you grow! *Circle all the things that grow, just like you do!*

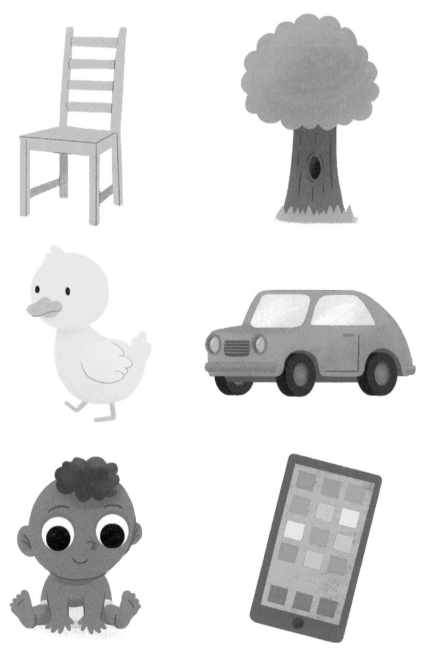

Breathing to the Beat!

Your lungs breathe in air to get oxygen. The oxygen goes into your blood and your heart pumps all that blood around your body. *Complete the maze to help the kid blow up the balloon.*

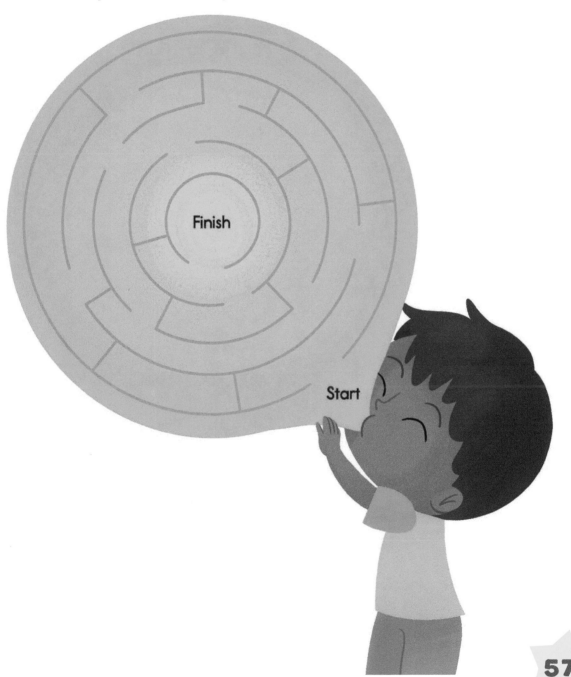

Finish

Start

Good Communication

Your brain and nerves send messages all over your body. Your body also sends messages back to your brain! *Connect the dots to complete the brain!*

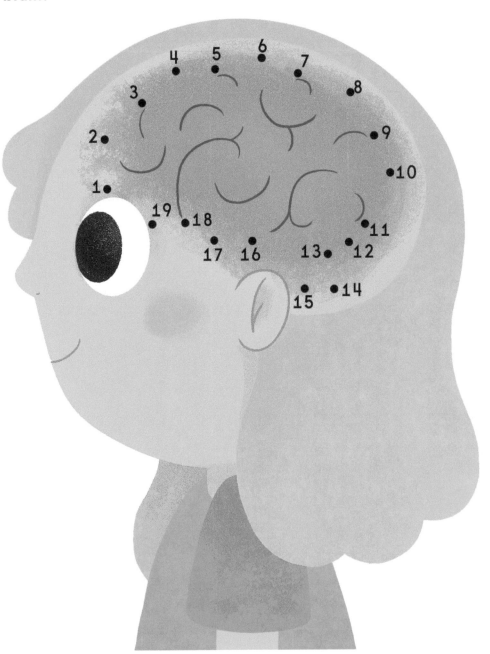

Natural Defense

Your immune system has a lot of parts that keep you healthy. Its job is to fight germs and keep you from getting sick! *Color the germs in all different colors!*

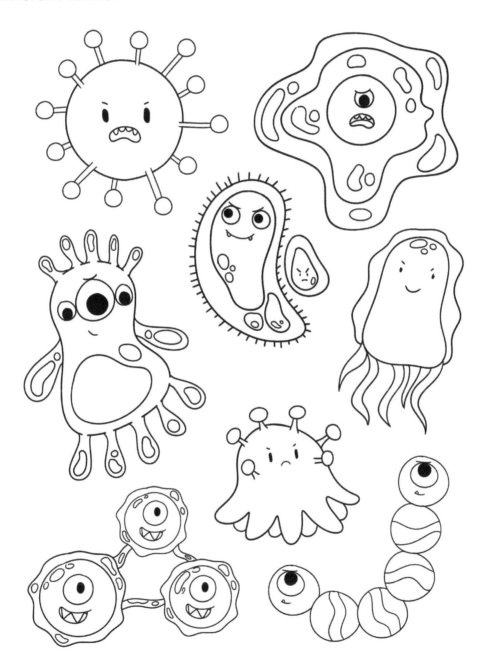

Team Body!

All of your body parts work together to keep you healthy and growing strong. *Finish the picture of the kid celebrating their body. Then jump up and celebrate yours, too!*

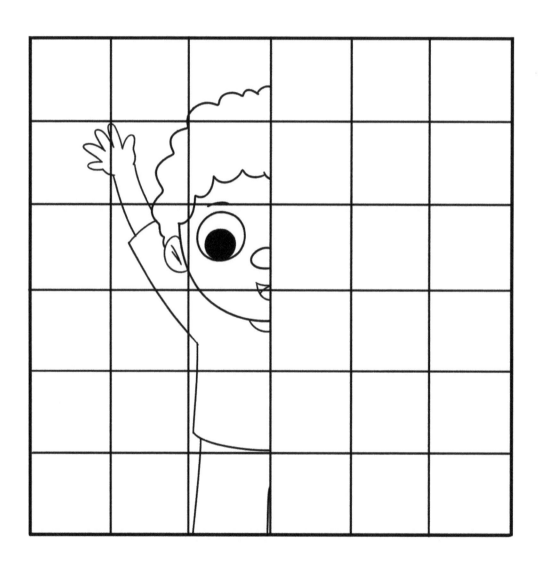

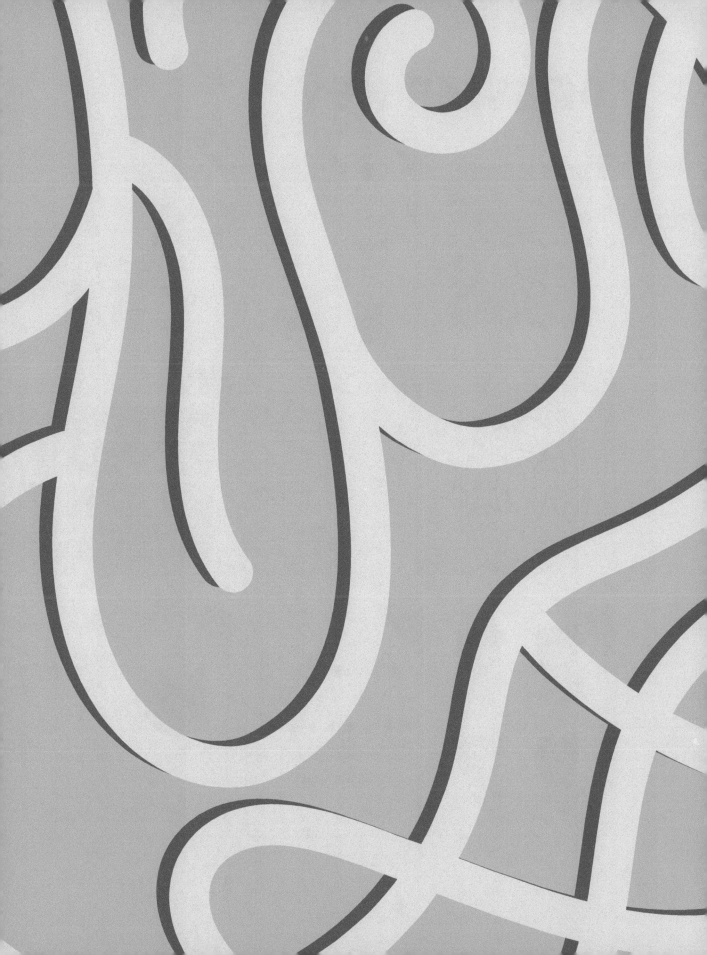

ANSWER KEY

1

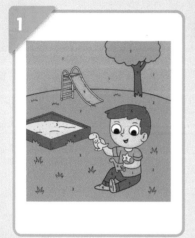

2

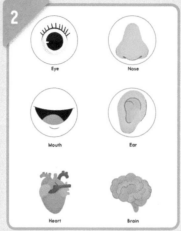

Eye Nose

Mouth Ear

Heart Brain

4

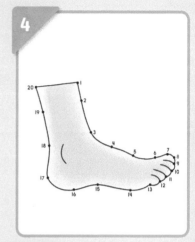

5

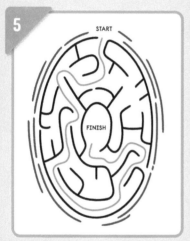

START

FINISH

6

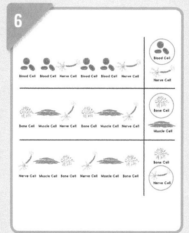

Blood Cell Blood Cell Nerve Cell Blood Cell Blood Cell Nerve Cell Blood Cell

Nerve Cell

Bone Cell Muscle Cell Nerve Cell Bone Cell Muscle Cell Nerve Cell Bone Cell

Muscle Cell

Nerve Cell Muscle Cell Bone Cell Nerve Cell Muscle Cell Bone Cell Bone Cell

Nerve Cell

8

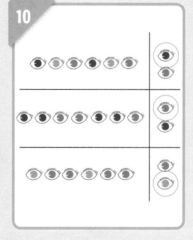

9

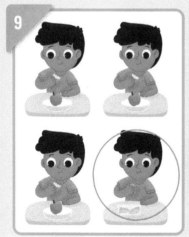

10

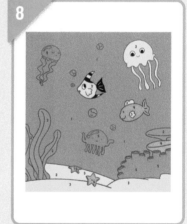

11

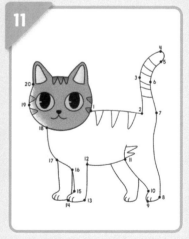

12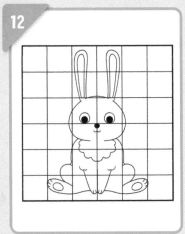

14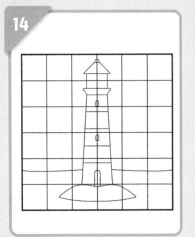

15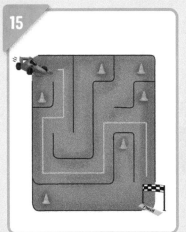

16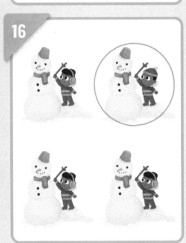

17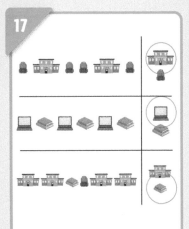

19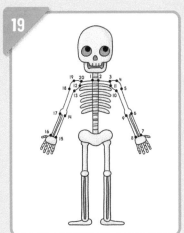

20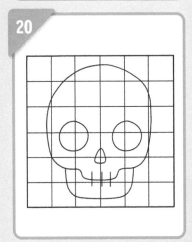

21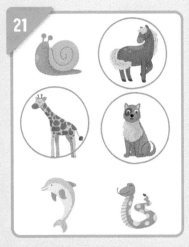

22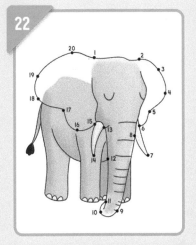

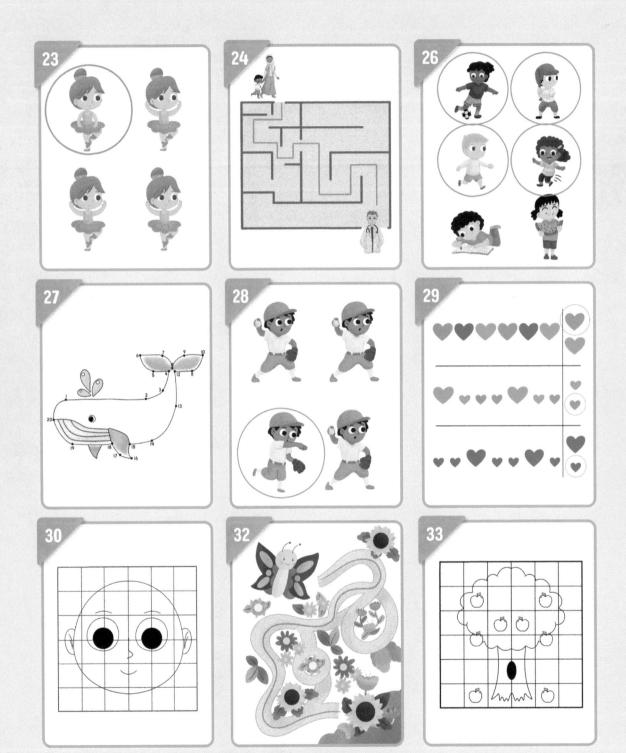

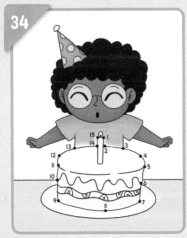

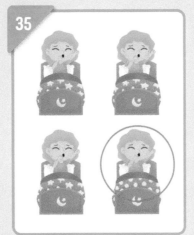

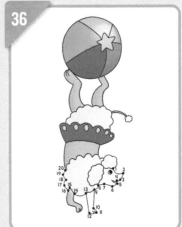

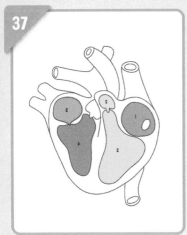

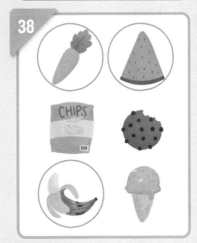

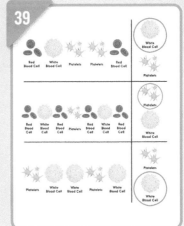

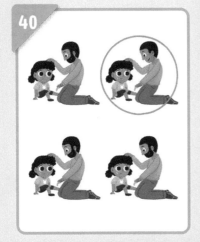

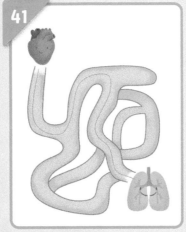

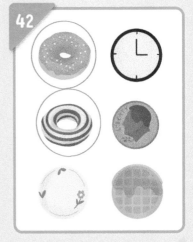

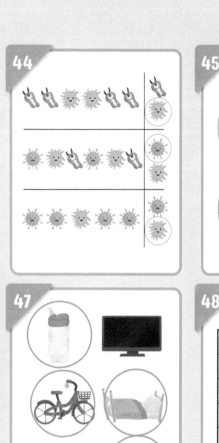

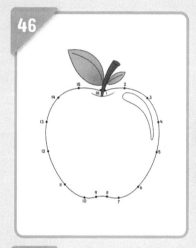

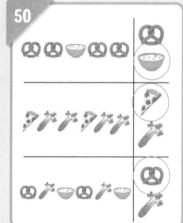

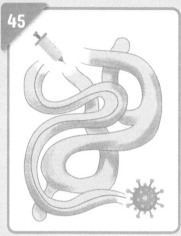

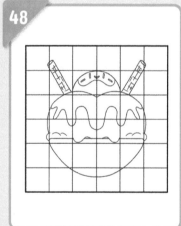

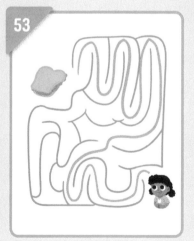

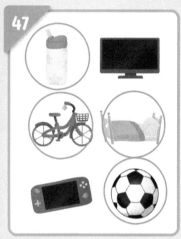

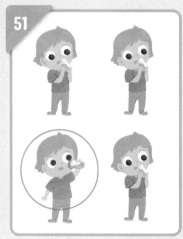

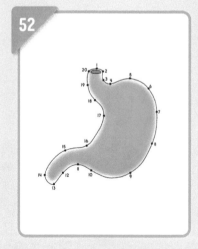

54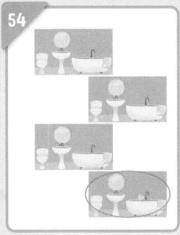

56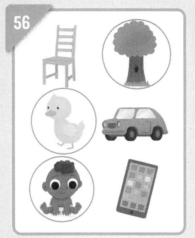

57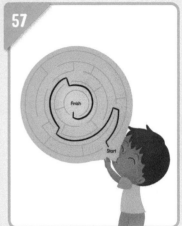

58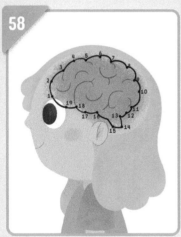

60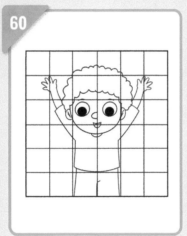

About the Author

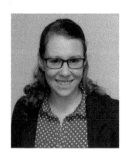

KRISTIE WAGNER is a middle-high school science teacher in southeast Wisconsin. She previously taught five years of high school science, one year of middle school science, and has a master of science in ecological teaching and learning. In her teaching career, she has designed curriculum for Physical Science (for grades 8 and 10), Biology (grades 9 and 10), Advanced Biology (grade 12), Anatomy and Physiology (grade 11), and Environmental Science (grades 11 and 12). Kristie currently works on a climate change education team creating and reviewing content for the North American Association for Environmental Education, which she has done since 2019. She is also the author of *Human Anatomy for Kids: A Junior Scientist's Guide to How We Move, Breathe, and Grow*. She lives with her husband and sons near a nature preserve. She loves to hike, nature journal, and read. She always finds resources to help her keep learning new things!